MY LITTLE PEOPLE

A HOSPICE SOCIAL WORKER'S JOURNEY

By Annie Clara Brown

My Little People
A Hospice Social Worker's Journey
All Rights Reserved.

ISBN-13: 9798656743617
Also in eBook edition

Copyright © 2020 Annie Clara Brown

All rights reserved. No part of this book may be reproduced in any form or by electronic or mechanical means, including information storage and retrieval systems, without permission in writing from the author, except by a reviewer who may quote brief passages in a review.

Cover Image © Pezibear_Pixabay
Cover & Interior Design by The Author's Mentor,
www.theauthorsmentor.com
A Division of
www.littleronipublishers.com

Author Website: https://bysttt.net

PUBLISHED IN THE UNITED STATES OF AMERICA

Dedication

This book is dedicated to all of the people who have allowed me to walk into their homes, hold their hands, cry with them, pray with them, help access resources, and allowed me to be part of their families. The names have been changed to protect their identity.

I must warn you some of these stories will make you laugh and some cry. There will be times when you will reflect on your own experiences and how some of these stories are similar.

I hope and pray that some of you will grow in your faith and that if there is anyone in your family who has wronged you that you will forgive them and if you have wronged others, then ask for forgiveness.

Why did I make that prior statement about forgiveness? Simply put, none of us know where death is or what the day holds for each of us.

2020 Special Dedication to my son, Detrick Baker, who lost his battle with cancer.

Table of Contents

Preface 1
Part I 7
   Introduction to my Hospice Journey 9
   My Personal Experience 12
   After the Admission of a Patient: The Social Worker Gets Busy 19
   Self-Care Tips for Hospice Social workers, Caregivers, and Other Professionals 30
   Patient and Family Comforts 36
Part II 46
   The Question 47
   What's in a Name? 49
   Precious Memories Last a Lifetime: Wonderful Patient Tales 51
Part III 108
   Annie's Personal Rewards for Serving 109
   A Prayer I Will Not Soon Forget 114
   My Heart's Desire 116
About the Author 118

Preface

"Life is uncertain, but death is sure" is a saying that I heard many years before I started my professional journey in social work. Talking about death was always a bleak subject to me. Who wants to discuss death? Even though the Holy Scriptures speak much about the subject, it is not one of those subjects that the average person is comfortable about discussing. No matter how uncomfortable the subject of death maybe, the angel of death has visited all of our homes at some time in our lives. Even as I sit here typing someone is taking their last breath and a loved one is sad because of the loss. As long as there is a world and people inhabit the land, there will be death. Not only will there be death, but sickness will continue to end in death for many people. While God is a healer, it remains a mystery why some people with certain illnesses live longer and others die sooner. In the midst of the whys and how comes, many things we will not have an answer to until the return of Christ.

With the never ending advances in technology it would seem that there was some magical formula to prevent death, but there has been research and more research and yet death occurs. Death itself is not a new concept because death has been occurring since life and sin in the Garden of Eden. When reviewing Biblical history, it still amazes me how long some of the people lived in the Bible days, but yet eventually they died, with the exception of Enoch, who walked with God and one day he was gone / translated. As we have moved from generation to generation, we have learned new ways to take care of a person who has a terminal diagnosis and has been given a time limit on their life. When I was a child people died at home, but they did not have the comforts that have come into existence for people in the twentieth century. So what has changed? It is called hospice.

So what is this phenomenon called hospice? Sounds like a great new innovation and indeed it is; therefore, where did the concept come from?

According to National Hospice Foundation:

The inspiration for the modern hospice movement came from Dame Cicely Saunders, who as a student of nursing in her native England during World War II, witnessed a great deal of suffering and pain. She came to believe that three things were most important in easing life's final journey. People needed strong relief from physical pain and troublesome symptoms, they needed to preserve their dignity, and they needed help with the psychological and spiritual pain of death. After some years in the nursing profession, Dame Cicely obtained degrees in medicine and social work, and in 1967 she established St. Christopher's Hospice in London. Ever since its doors opened, St. Christopher's treatment philosophy has been to help individuals in the final stages of life live in dignity and comfort. Her approach involved a marriage of disciplines: pain management, emotional and spiritual support, and family counseling. The care was delivered by a team of medical and nursing professionals as well as social workers and spiritual counselors. Much gratitude goes to Dr. Saunders for having the courage to venture out into a field of practice that most people had no knowledge of.

A few years before Dr. Saunders opened St. Christopher's; she delivered a lecture at Yale University in New Haven about her ideas. That lecture helped launch hospice care in America, for among those in the audience was Florence Wald, then dean of Yale's School of Nursing. According to Wald, Dame Cicely's words changed the direction of her life. Wald left the deanship in 1968 and traveled to London where she worked at St. Christopher's hospice to learn its approach to patient care and to study the hospice's organization and management. Six years later, in 1974, with the help of two physicians, Florence Wald founded Connecticut Hospice in Branford, on the outskirts of New Haven. As the first hospice in the United States, it was also first to offer home care and today, throughout the country, over 90% of hospice care is delivered at home.

Since the mid-1970s when hospice care was introduced in America as the most innovative, comprehensive and humane care available for people with limited life expectancies; demand for hospice care has increased every year.

One of the most important developments in expanding access to quality end-of-life care was the passage of the Medicare Hospice Benefit in 1982, through which hospices receive federal funds for the care they give to eligible patients. With this legislation, the federal government essentially declared that hospice care was so important in relieving suffering and in bringing about a peaceful and meaningful closure to life, that every citizen was entitled to it, regardless of ability to pay. Although federal reimbursements for providing hospice care have fallen behind the real costs of this care, this benefit has nevertheless supported the growth of quality end-of-life care for all Americans. (National Hospice Foundation)

Part I

- ➢ Introduction to My Hospice Journey
- ➢ My Personal Experience
- ➢ After the Admission of a Patient: The Social Worker Gets Busy
- ➢ Self-Care Tips for Social Workers and Caregivers
- ➢ Patient and Family Comforts

Introduction to my Hospice Journey

Even at its onset, while hospice was a new way of taking care of people in their homes, it was not a strange phenomenon because even when I was born, physicians made house calls. However, today I am thankful for how the hospice concept caught on and expanded to my state of residence (Alabama). If hospice had not been successful and Alabama had not gotten into the hospice movement, I would not have received this remarkable opportunity to work in such a rewarding job. The insight from knowledgeable doctors, nurses, social workers, home health aides, office administrators, chaplains, and volunteers has added so much value to shaping me into the professional I have become today. However it has been the patients and their families who have enriched my life and helped me to grow to new depths and heights in maturing as a Christian with a heart full of thanks.

I am eternally grateful for all my learning experiences and the opportunities to serve this population of individuals and be invited into their lives at one of the most vulnerable times a person can experience. Needless to say I am proud to be called a medical social worker who works with the terminally ill.

So why do I consider it important to write a book on hospice care? One reason is that I believe it is important for social workers, patients, and caregivers to understand how rewarding it is to be able to assist families at one of the most critical times in their lives as the patient is preparing to make a transition from earth to eternity.

Another reason is that as the generation of baby boomers are aging and suffering from terminal diseases, there is going to be a greater need for compassionate social workers and other healthcare professionals to take care of us. Also patients' caregivers need to understand that they have help available to them so they do not have to take the journey alone. I have witnessed that having hospice in the home and being spared some of the stress of trying to get the patient to a doctor's appointment or go for tests is invaluable.

Finally, in earlier years, I was a caregiver for several of my family members who suffered from a terminal illness and I had no idea that the option was available to have my family members cared for at home; therefore, it is my personal mission to help educate others about such a vital service to patients and their families. In hindsight, if only I had known some of the following information, some of the wear and tear on my body and unnecessary trips late at night to the hospital could have been avoided. I did not know, but I want you (the readers) to know.

My Personal Experience

In my life, as stated previously, I have had many losses as the result of death from terminal illnesses as I am sure many of you have also, or will have in the future. Since being educated about the services provided by hospice, in hindsight, I wish that I'd had hospice with my mother when she was diagnosed with colon cancer. My mother was transferred back and forth to doctor's offices and the hospital as needs arose. She spent her last days before her death in a hospital. Knowing what I know today, I wish I could go back in time; I would have helped my mother stay in the comfort of her home with the help of hospice care.

To have quality care in the home during a terminal illness I have found is so beneficial. Not having to be exposed to constant needle pricks, being awakened in the middle of the night to have your temperature taken, long trips to the doctor's office, and test after test being performed with the same prognosis of death, when a loved one could be at home comfortable is so much more humane.

How do I make the decision to get hospice involved or how do I know when to call in hospice?

I hear individuals say so often, "I just had a physical, but soon after the physical I just was not feeling well; therefore, I went to see my doctor and he/she ran some tests and now he/she is telling me I am dying. So what do I do? If I take radiation or chemo therapy it is not going to help me, according to scientific evidence. My prognosis is that I have six months or less to live if the disease process follows its normal progression."

Question after question begins to come to mind like: What do I do? Where do I turn for help? Many people have explained, "I want to be as comfortable as I can be, I want to maintain my dignity, and at the same time I want to be surrounded by my family and friends and not have to be in a clinical setting like a hospital." Hopefully, you have heard about hospice, because this is when you need to start to thinking about hospice care and which agency you want to provide services to your loved one or yourself. Researching hospices is always recommended, but at times there is not enough time for research. One of the greatest advertising tools is "word of mouth." There should be someone you personally know who has used hospice before or ask your primary physician.

While there will always be those who have had positive experiences with hospice, we have to understand that there are also the negative experiences. With the knowledge that hospice is like any other business, people need to understand their rights. An important fact to know is that you have a choice of which hospice you want you or your loved ones to use. Just because your doctor recommends a certain hospice service, doesn't mean you have to use it; if you know of another hospice you would prefer, then speak up and let your doctor know that. It might be the case that after a hospice agency is in your home, the services might not meet your needs or expectations; remember, you still have the right to change services if you desire to do so.

Where are these services provided?

These services can be provided in the comfort of where you reside. In times like these I hope that you and your family have been made aware of hospice and understand the hospice concept for end of life care. If you do not have a working knowledge of hospice, please contact your local hospice office and ask questions. Since you are reading this book you will have a jump start on most people, because I will give you some concepts of what services hospice provides. Even though the concepts listed are not all inclusive because regulations change often, you will still have a general idea of what's available. Above all, it is my desire that if the need arises in your life, you will not hesitate to call on hospice to assist you through your difficult time with a terminal illness.

Where can I live and be provided hospice care?

Hospice services can be provided in the comfort of your own home, nursing home, with family members, general inpatient in the hospital, inpatient hospice, or wherever you live out your last days. With the exception of if you live in a facility that is considered unlicensed, such as certain assisted living homes and boarding homes, because the public health department deems it is not permissible to enter to care for patients due to the absence of regulatory mandates. To enter these facilities means we would be breaking state or federal laws.

What are some of the services generally provided by hospice care?

Some of the services are as follows:
- Home visits by specialty trained hospice nurses and Medical Director

- Pain management and symptom control
- Personal hygiene care from certified home health aides
- All medications related to the terminal diagnosis
- All specialized therapies required for the terminal diagnosis
- Psychosocial, spiritual, and grief support services
- Volunteers as requested

What is the role of a social worker in hospice care with respect to case management?

Most of the services listed above, a social worker does not have the training to perform. As with any professional discipline, social workers must stay within their scope of practice. In many organizations social workers are considered to be case managers; however, in hospice, nurses serve in the role of case managers. And rightly so because they have the responsibility of making decisions as to what care plans are best for each patient when it comes to medications, symptoms management, and daily visits. Of course a hospice nurse does so much more, but that is the general idea of what a nurse does.

I mentioned that aspect of hospice because in most settings the social worker is considered to be the case manager. Many times it takes some adjusting for a social worker to work in a hospice environment and not be expected to take the lead. However, when the roles are clearly defined, there is no doubt who is the leader of the team for each patient. Teamwork keeps everything flowing smoothly and boundaries are vital.

After the Admission of a Patient: The Social Worker Gets Busy

So what do social workers do in hospice? I cannot say what roles all social workers fill, but I can give a general idea of what my day is like. When considering every family and their dynamics are unique, there is no set rule on what I do for any one family; it just depends on their needs and what can be done to make life a little less stressful. No person should have to sit by their loved one's bedside worrying about a utility bill or food.

While this is hard for some to believe, there are still families in our country who are poor. For these families their greatest resource is their love for one another. It seems that in our great nation that lack would not be an issue; but believe me, poverty is still alive and well. I need to make a vital point here: *While finding resources for caregivers and patients is not a role that is exclusive to hospice social workers, finding resources in a timely manner is.*

As a social worker, helping others is one of our greatest assets. Social workers are looked upon as "knowing" what resources are available. After ten years in hospice I continue to value staying informed about current available resources. Some states have more resources than others, so each year it would be helpful to research which resources are available year after year and what is new. Attending workshops in your area about resources is vital. I really appreciate the hard work done by the United Way in establishing 211 which is a nationwide resource that can be used to ask about resources wherever you live.

I have chosen to highlight typical family needs for prospective hospice social workers to address when conducting an initial psychosocial assessment. The hospice team also depends on the social worker to provide at a moment's notice the emotional support each family needs to make the care in the home go as smooth as can be.

The following is preliminary information to address when completing a psychosocial on a patient:

1. A responsible caregiver is always needed to provide care for the patient. Many times when a person is admitted, he/she may be up and walking around but we know without divine intervention, a decline will come. Therefore, at some point the patient will need another person to take on the role of a caregiver. No two persons are the same and the degree of care needed will be different. However, one thing that is certain is sooner most times than later, a decline will begin and the patient will need more and more care from someone other than themselves. It is vital that this decision is in place to have someone in charge to be able to carry out the duties needed. Why? Because bedbound

patients with terminal illnesses reach a point when they are not safe if not supervised. Some are fall risks, susceptible to confusion and cannot take medications appropriately, have pain crises, many smokers endanger themselves falling asleep and dropping lit cigarettes, and many forget they are wearing oxygen and just light up cigarettes. Safety education is always in order.

2. The age range for hospice patients varies. Since this is the case it is important to explain the need for legal paperwork, for example: living wills/advanced directives, powers of attorney, last will and testaments and also bank accounts beneficiaries. This is also important for people who do not have a terminal illness it just makes good business sense for anybody.

3. Anyone who is 19 years old (in Alabama) and is competent can express their wishes for what they prefer in reference to their healthcare. This may not apply to every state because age for

decision making can vary. Many people shy away from talking about this but every family needs to have "the talk." The talk is not something you will need to do over and over again but someone in the family needs to know what you want if there comes a time when you will not be able to make a medical decision on your own because you are terminal or have some kind of accident that leaves you incapable of making decisions. Verbal consent is fine, but written instructions are better; hence the need for a living will or advanced directive. In that discussion, you will need to make plain your preference of Do Not Resuscitate (DNR), which means when your heart stops, do you want anyone pumping on your chest trying to get your heart started back, or not. It is your choice. It is good to have a full understanding of DNR and Do Not Intubate (DNI) because at that moment when death is imminent, time is of the essence. Do not intubate means that you want someone performing chest compressions (CPR) but do not want to be kept alive by a machine after being revived. It is also good to realize that when the patient is dying in the home, there is not the required equipment available to keep organs in healthy condition until organs can be harvested by an Organ Removal Team. Therefore organ donations are mostly limited to the eyes; however, there is the option for body donation for research.

4. A Power of attorney is responsible for taking care of the patient's financial obligations such as paying his/her bills and purchasing items needed. With privacy policies in place, it is virtually impossible to obtain any information on another person without legal authority. Make sure that you consider this if you decide you might not need a power of attorney. Even husbands and wives need legal authority in writing to get health care and other vital information about each other. Let me give you an example of what I am talking about. Say, for instance, Mrs. Right needs some information on Mr. Right from a doctor, bank, loan, or phone bill and Mrs. Right is not listed on

the accounts, guess what they will not even tell you if Mr. Right is a patient or client. Sounds silly, right? Well, silly or not, Mr. Right's medical information and bills are protected by the privacy act. One of my patients' wives died and neither he nor anyone else was listed on her bank account. Guess what? After her death, my patient needed the money in the bank to help with her funeral and he could not touch that money until after a long, drawn-out procedure mandated by law. This is just one of the things I have experienced and want others not to have to go through. Last will and testaments are vital because a power of attorney, if in place, dies with the patient. It is always good to put on paper what you want others to do and have of yours after you are dead and gone.

5. Ask about funeral plans for the patient. It is always good to know how to assist the patient and their families. Too many people are dying and leaving family members, who are already in emotional pain, to stress about resources to bury a

loved one. It is important to have some kind of frame of reference of what a patient's and their family's preference is about funerals, burials or cremations. While the lack of funds or insurance to pay the expenses is a special consideration when planning a funeral/cremation, it is also wise to know about cultural beliefs. If you do not know the particulars, then make it your business to find out what others want, because everyone is entitled to their choices. Many choose to leave a legacy by using their bodies to further medical research. Your loved one's body can be donated for research, if certain eligibility requirements are met.

6. Many patients who come to hospice are indigent. Indigent does not always mean that a person does not have resources, but rather that they do not have a healthcare insurance source to pay for hospice services. As I mentioned earlier, time is of the essence. Lining up resources for a family is crucial. It is important that a social worker know about such resources as…

- Social Security Benefits are available to most disabled persons. A person's work history and meeting certain criteria will determine if a person is eligible for Social Security Disability (SSD) or Supplemental Security Income (SSI).
- Veteran Benefits are dependent on meeting certain criteria for benefits as set forth by the Veteran's Administration. Community resources for helping with various needs, such as Meals on Wheels or power/gas assistance.
- Cancer insurance policies for people with a cancer diagnosis can be a great resource when money is tight.
- Long–term care insurance is valuable when caregiving is needed and hiring others outside of the family is required.
- Life Insurance, while it is good to have after a person has died, it can also be useful while a person is alive, if there is an accelerated death benefit attached. Many times families just do not have the ability to leave their jobs for long periods of time but when an accelerated benefit

is attached to a policy, up to half of that policy benefit can be used to help with a terminally ill patient's care before he/she dies.

- FMLA (Family Medical Leave Act) is a good resource for caregivers if their employers provide it. A person can take up to twelve weeks off work to care for their loved ones.

7. Even though continuing education is a requirement for licensure purposes, it is also an important way for social workers to stay on top of changes that may affect their ability to help patients and their families.

While the above list of documents and resources are addressed by social workers during a psychosocial assessment and every attempt will be made to assist the patient and their families, it is not always feasible. Therefore; it is very important that each family already have these documents on hand because when hospice comes on board, more often than not there is not enough time to get these documents in place. Regrettably, sometimes the patient's mental status does not allow him/her to be competent enough to take care of the task of getting these documents signed and notarized. Of course when it comes to a power of attorney and the patient is not competent enough to make decisions for him or herself, there is another legal option of getting a judge to appoint the patient a guardian or conservator. Of course the above list is not all inclusive of the services a hospice social worker provides, but it is a great starting point and more tips will be given in the second part of my journey.

Self-Care Tips for Hospice Social workers, Caregivers, and Other Professionals

Some of the issues social workers or caregivers experience can be heart wrenching; therefore, it is just as important for social workers and caregivers to take care of themselves as they care for others. Most social workers/caregivers try to be fixers, but we cannot fix anyone but ourselves, although we can offer suggestions.

One of my quotes I use for caregivers is applicable for social workers, "You cannot care for your loved ones if you do not take care of yourself." Since caregivers are with the patient more than anyone else, it is vital that caregivers find a way to take care of themselves. It is important to remember that as a caregiver you cannot be everything to everybody and not become exhausted. Allow others to help. Further tips will be given for caregivers in the second part of this journey.

Many skills are learned in the school of social work and then there are lessons that are learned from experience. Over the years, I have been asked to teach other social workers some of the things that make a good social worker. While I can share some skills, there are some things that are innate and cannot be taught because they come directly from God. It is my belief that every social worker who works in the healthcare field of hospice should have a personal relationship with God. Why? As a social worker you might be the person who will be given the honor of leading a person to Christ before they take their last breath.

With that being said, let us continue this journey with some "suggestions" that I have found to be very helpful for me as a social worker that are applicable to both social workers and caregivers.

- ✓ **Always stay true to yourself.** You should understand your beliefs and know your own biases. Decisions are made from our frame of reference and can be a shortcoming if we do not understand what we believe and how our beliefs determine how we view a situation. There is no place for being judgmental.
- ✓ **Always be willing to listen.** No one is right all the time and as social workers, caregivers, and other professionals, we have to be willing to be open-minded. Our way is not always the right way or the only way to resolve a situation. Seek counsel from more experienced workers to get clarity when unsure. It is best to ask for help rather than try to prove a point.
- ✓ **Don't take everything personally.** The best of individuals have bad days and if someone speaks sharply to you or ignores you, it does not mean it is personal toward you. Give others the benefit of the doubt, because we

do not always know what others are being confronted with. Rest assured you will need the same compassion at some time or other.

- ✓ **Know your limitations.** No one is an expert on every topic, so if you do not know an answer it is alright. Be willing to acknowledge that you do not have the answer, but be determined to find an appropriate answer. People know when we are not truthful and faking; this can hurt what could have become a trusting relationship.
- ✓ **Be a team player.** The most important person is the patient. Consult with team and family members to seek the best way to help a patient. By all means if the patient is able to participate, include him/her in decision making. What worked for one patient and family may not work for others and the other team members who have interacted with the patient/family may have some insight into how to find a resolution that we have not

considered. Many times when providing comfort care, disciplines cross over into other disciplines.

- ✓ **Be prayerful.** Seeking the wisdom of God is always in order. If we acknowledge God, He will direct our paths. Sometimes we are just at a loss and we want to help, but nothing we do seems to be right no matter how hard we try.
- ✓ **Be thankful.** No matter what your own situation is, it could be worse. Positions could be reversed to where we would be the one needing understanding. But if we want understanding we have to give it.
- ✓ **Be willing to give.** The best social workers are those who will go the extra mile to find a resource or provide support to a patient/family. Sometimes you have to do things off the clock and do them willingly. Social work is a profession that serves. But know your limits.

- ✓ **Be an advocate.** Regardless of how good a patient's intentions are to make decisions on his/her own it is not always possible. When a patient/family is in harm's way in terms of neglect, abuse, suicide, etc., we have to be willing to intervene. Of course we want patients/families to be able to exercise self-determination; however, that is not always possible. Know when to make a referral.
- ✓ **Recognize burnout.** Working with hospice is one of the most rewarding areas of social work that I can think of; however, when we start to feel that it is just a job and we fail to care about people, it is time we reassess. Not everyone is suited for the continual pressures of the job.

Patient and Family Comforts

The following are some of the comforts that are available for patients and families when questions come up.

Spiritual Care

Spiritual care at the end of life is as important for comfort measures as physical care. Many patients and their families rely on their faith to help them through the process of a terminal illness. I am a firm believer that trusting God to be there to lean on is of great value. Every hospice is responsible for the spiritual care of the patient and their families as needed.

I have heard many testimonies of how the prayers of the chaplains, nurses and, of course, social workers have helped patients and families. That is what is so phenomenal about working with patients in hospice; if a chaplain is not available to provide prayer at a particular time, then nurses, home health aides, volunteers, or the social worker can step into the role to provide comfort through prayer and scriptures while in the home as needed or requested.

Knowing the deep hurt that comes with loss, spiritual care is a major component of palliative care at the end of life. It is my desire that every patient who comes to death's door will know God so that God can carry them on into Paradise.

Bereavement

Since everyone grieves differently and grief is unique to every individual, it is important for a hospice team, especially chaplains and social workers, to understand the many kinds of grief there are. Many books have been written about the process of grief and there continues to be debates about the stages of grief that Elisabeth Kübler-Ross penned. Nevertheless, one thing is certain and that is it hurts when we experience the loss of a loved one and sometimes we do not know how to react. Therefore, I am of the opinion that there is not any certain formula for how a person is supposed to show their grief.

From my own personal experience with loss, I find that grief is much like dancing the waltz or cha-cha where persons move backwards and forward. Many times we think we have made several steps in what we perceive is the right direction and suddenly there is a trigger and it feels like we are back to the day we first experienced the loss. There are many factors to take into consideration when grieving. Every loss is different. It also depends on the dynamics of the relationship with the person who died that dictates the steps a person will go through and how long it will be that the grief is all that you can feel. Many times grief becomes complicated and there is a need to seek professional help, especially when all you can feel is grief and you are unable to move past the initial grief.

The Center for Complicated Grief, describes complicated grief as follows:

Complicated grief is an intense and long-lasting form of grief that takes over a person's life. It is natural to experience acute grief after someone close dies, but complicated grief is different. Complicated grief takes hold of a person's mind and won't let go. People with complicated grief often say that they feel "stuck."

For most people, grief never completely goes away but recedes into the background. Over time, healing diminishes the pain of a loss. Thoughts and memories of loved ones are deeply interwoven in a person's mind, defining their history and coloring their view of the world.

Missing deceased loved ones may be an ongoing part of the lives of bereaved people, but it does not interrupt life unless a person is suffering from complicated grief. For people suffering with complicated grief, grief takes over their lives rather than moving into the background. Since complicated grief is becoming more prevalent, I would like to share a definition of complicated grief from a reliable source other than myself that I have found helpful.

This source is also from the Center of Complicated Grief from Columbia University of Social Work. They write:

The term "complicated" refers to factors that interfere with the natural healing process. These factors might be related to characteristics of the bereaved person, to the nature of the relationship with the deceased person, the circumstances of the death, or to things that occurred after the death. People with complicated grief know their loved one is gone, but they still can't believe it. They say that time is moving on but they are not. They often have strong feelings of yearning or longing for the person who died that don't seem to lessen as time goes on. Thoughts, memories, or images of the deceased person frequently fill their mind, capturing their attention. They might have strong feelings of bitterness or anger related to the death. They find it hard to imagine that life without the deceased person has purpose or meaning. It can seem like joy and satisfaction are gone forever.

However, you can move forward with the right counsel and support.

Another kind of grief that many people tend to beat themselves up about is the grief that most refer to as anticipatory grief.

Anticipatory grief is what happens when you know there will be a loss, but it has not yet occurred. This is what happens when a loved one is dying, and both the patient and their loved ones have time to prepare. Anticipatory grief is both the easiest and the hardest kind of grief to experience. It is marked by "stop and go" signals. With these losses, the handwriting is on the wall... but it doesn't make coping with it easier.

Because you have time to prepare, you can begin to envision and rehearse your life without the person who is dying. This gift of time offers the opportunity to resolve any regrets you may have with or about your loved one. You can take this time to make amends with your loved one, and to tell him or her how you feel about them. Your loved one can do the same with you, and other family members. You can let go of anger or guilt. You also have the chance for delicate conversations about such sensitive topics as death, end of life wishes, and after-death preparation. You also have an opportunity to get information about your family.

One obvious drawback to anticipatory grief is witnessing your loved one's struggle with death. As the loved one's condition worsens, you may grieve with each downturn. You may experience feeling a sense of helplessness as your loved one fights for life. You may feel as if you are living with a pit in your stomach that won't go away as you await death's arrival. In addition, sometimes when people are facing death, their own fear, pain, or anger may make their personality seem to change from Dr. Jekyll to Mr. Hyde overnight or even from one moment to the next. In my own case, when cancer took over my mother's body, she did not experience some of the confusion like others I have witnessed. I am forever grateful for that. But for some families, the ones we love continue to have behavioral changes as they face the end of life. This can be challenging, and having hospice care in the home to provide emotional support during this time can be comforting.

Perhaps the most difficult challenge with anticipatory grief is that it is difficult to tolerate living in a state of emergency for an extended period of time. The mind can only tolerate so much anguish. When a loved one is dying, the "emergency" and anxiety period may seem to last forever. You do not want your loved one's death to come more quickly, yet your mind may not be able to handle when the process is prolonged. Your mind may blank out self-protectively.

But eventually, a reminder or a new episode with the loved one sets off the grief again. Here, intense grief comes in waves alternating with times of numbness. These "stop and go" signals allow you to shut down emotionally. This insulates you before the next event occurs. Then, your grief begins anew. These flat periods can be looked at as natural, normal, and a welcome respite from the agony of the loss. They do not mean you are cold or uncaring.

Anticipatory grief is normal. It is an important part of coping with a loved one's extended illness. It prepares both you and your loved one for the end of life. Unfortunately, it may also be an emotional roller coaster. If you can expect that and understand that, you can help yourself cope with it. Don't feel guilty about anything you may be feeling. Instead, make the best of each moment you can spend with your loved one, and focus on the positives, such as forgiveness, settling affairs, and helping your loved one make plans for their passing.

Both complicated and anticipatory grief was mentioned because they are the two kinds of grief that have people questioning their sanity. After the death of a loved one, when anticipatory grief is experienced, I often hear that the person is not so overwhelmed because he/she grieved the loss while the person was living. Whether this is what you may go through; yet again, depend on the dynamics surrounding the end of life circumstances. Many times the loss is experienced at such a rapid rate that there is not time for anticipatory grief.

Hospice families should not be left to manage their grief alone after death therefore the hospice agency provides bereavement follow up for a year. Another service that goes under bereavement is grief support. Grief Support is not only provided for the adults but for children and adolescents. When possible it is suggested that children and adolescents be part of the dying process with their loved ones. Children have the tendency to grieve differently than adults but we must remember we cannot protect them from the reality of death and dying. Death is part of life and we all have to experience it at some stage in life; regretfully, some younger than others.

Part II

- ✓ The Question
- ✓ What's in a Name?
- ✓ Precious Memories Last a Lifetime: Wonderful Patient Tales

The Question

Someone once asked me, "Do you get depressed every day when dealing with people with terminal illnesses?" I answered sincerely and told him no. Of course there are those who I become more attached to than others and I feel sadness. I cry if I must, but many times after watching the decline of a patient, when death finally comes I feel relief that the suffering is over. When a person has glorified God in life then when death comes, sometimes I feel a little spiritual jealousy because they are with Jesus and I am left to face the evil created by people still alive.

I feel so rich that I have been able to share some of the most precious moments with people from all walks of life. Each person has a story to tell and I love to hear them: stories of failures, accomplishments, ups and downs, wars, love, peace, grace, travels, etc. It is because I have been so blessed that I want to share the wealth. So let us embark on a journey as we take a lovely stroll through some of my more memorable patients' lives as I interacted with them.

What's in a Name?

"Your little people, your little people, you always have to go see your little people." Mrs. H was a patient with dementia who was a joy to visit in her home. She loved the color red and she loved people. Mrs. H. would always ask me when I visited, "Where have you been?" She was not oriented to time; therefore, she always perceived that each visit had been a long time off; however, my visits were made every two weeks. One day, when she asked where I had been, I replied that I had been visiting my little people. She began to speak in a mimicking voice, "Your little people, your little people, you always have to go see your little people."

From that day on, this was basically how she acknowledged me when I visited. After she said the magic words (your little people, your little people, you always have to go see your little people), most of the time she would drift off into confusion. One day she thought the leaves on the trees outside her window had faces on them. I always smile when I hear the phrase your little people because memories of Mrs. H. come to mind. May she rest in peace.

Precious Memories Last a Lifetime: Wonderful Patient Tales

The most precious persons in hospice are the patients. These individuals invite hospice workers into their homes at one of the most critical times in their lives. A loved one has received some devastating news and that news has turned their world inside out. Regardless of the dynamics of the diagnosis, what is foremost in the minds of their loved ones is the prognosis and the fact that unless an Almighty God in His infinite wisdom decides that He will divinely heal, then, death will be the result. It was when dealing with one of these dear patients that the idea was birthed to write about my journey with hospice. Careful thought is always given to a book's name and it was no less with the name of this book. Who would have thought that a precious moment with a patient and her mocking me would be the result of a title of a book? I know you are going to fall in love with these dear hearts as I tell of my experiences with some of them. So enjoy!

Mr. A:
God's Grace and Mercy Met Me at the Door

Mr. A was 102 when I met him. I went to his residence and he answered the door. I was expecting this person at the door to take me to see the patient. When he identified himself as the patient, I was taken aback. As I began to conduct my assessment, I continued to wait on this man to start rambling in confusion or become disoriented because he was 102, but it never happen. Actually, confusion and disorientation only came a couple of weeks before his transition to heaven.

Mr. A loved God and to hear him talk about God and God's saving grace was truly a life changing experience. Sometimes Mr. A would become tearful in his praise and thanksgiving for God's saving grace. Mr. A was unique in that he did not believe that you retired from your service to God. When he was unable to preach in the pulpit, Mr. A and his wife had a daily devotion and prayer time in their home. They had a prayer list that they prayed over daily.

Let me tell you about Mr. A and his wife. Mr. A's first wife had died and Mr. A married his second wife who had been a friend of Mr. A and his first wife. Mr. A and his second wife had been married for eleven years when I came into the picture. They were the perfect picture of what a married couple should be. They were always exchanging endearments of sweetheart and darling. On one occasion, Mrs. A had burned some biscuits and Mr. A used a scriptural text to explain the issue. Mr. A stated that Mrs. A had given him a burnt offering that day. We had the biggest laugh and often when I visited I would ask if he'd had another burnt offering.

While visiting with Mr. A one day he began to talk about going to heaven. He said that he used to have pall-bearers picked out to carry his casket. He stated that some of his remaining friends told him not to ask them to be a pall-bearer because every previous set of pall-bearers had died. I also told him not to invite me to his funeral because he might outlive me. What a joy to be able to laugh and see 'threescore and ten and by reason of strength' according to Psalm 90:20 lived out in reality.

It was so funny, on one occasion when some of Mr. A's great grandchildren were visiting that Mrs. A went out and purchased a ball so that she and the children could play. Mind you, Mrs. A was age eighty-nine. When I asked how that visit went she said she was disappointed that the children chose not to play ball, but instead sat at Mr. A's feet and wrote about Mr. A's history in his native land.

The most precious thing I experienced was having this great man of God pray for me and the staff of people that I worked with. Mr. A gave praise, glory, and thanks to God until he went home to be with his precious Savior, our Lord Jesus Christ.

Ms. S: Portrait of Love Through the Mind of a Woman/Child

Rarely does a person get to experience the love of an individual who was diagnosed from birth with a disability. I will not mention the name of the disability for identification purposes. The love of these individuals is so unconditional, though. My first encounter with Ms. S was when the hospice that I worked for took care of Ms. S's mother. Ms. S was one of those people that you fell in love with instantly. Her child-like personality made you want to protect her.

I remember going to her home and I introduced myself and she asked, "Are you married?" My reply was "no" and she stated "Me neither." I would tease her about her duties in the home. I would ask, "Do you cook?" and she would reply "no." She was not allowed to cook but she loved to eat and her favorite foods were Tacos and chocolate. It was so heartwarming to hear Ms. S talk about her mother, who she called "Precious."

Precious died. Several years afterwards, Ms. S. became my patient. This was one of my harder experiences but the most rewarding thing was the privileges of taking care of Ms. S. She did not have many good days, but on a good day when I visited, it brought so much joy to my heart. Ms. S, Ms. S's sister-in-law, and I had a secret. The secret was that Ms. S. supposedly had a boyfriend, but she did not want her brother, who was her caregiver, to know about her boyfriend. So when we attempted to talk about her boyfriend, she would put her little finger to her mouth so we would be quiet; however, she was not shy about letting everyone know that one day she was going to get married and she was going to have two children. She was not sure what to name one of the children, but she stated that she was going to name one, Billy Graham. She loved to watch Billy Graham on the television. One of her favorite sayings was, "Don't you get started."

A very memorable time with Ms. S and her family was hilarious. Ms. S's brother and sister-in-law had a dog. Ms. S called the dog "Buddy." We had a great laugh with Ms. S eldest brother because Ms. S became angry with him and would not speak to him for a long period of time because her brother called Buddy a dog. Everybody knew after that not to call the dog nothing but Buddy or you experienced Ms. S's wrath.

There is something special about a child-like spirit in an individual and though Ms. S was older in age than I was, she reminded me that at any age to love unconditionally is a gift. Ms. S died and went to heaven to be with her father and Precious. My life is so much richer because of knowing such a wonderful woman/child.

Mr. H:
Mistaken Identity

The care team for hospice has chaplains. So was the story of a Chaplain (Tom Simic) whose identity was mistaken for a movie star. Mr. H was a patient and his wife had problems pronouncing names. While visiting with Mrs. H. she informed me that she could not remember a chaplain (Tom Simic) last name; therefore she started to call him, Tom Selleck. After, Mr. H's death, I attended visitation for Mr. H, Chaplain (Tom Simic) had been to the funeral home before I had arrived. When I arrived, Mrs. H was standing with friends and she stated to me that Tom Selleck had been there earlier.

The ladies having experienced firsthand how tired Mrs. H had been when caring for Mr. H, appeared to think that Mrs. H was having a moment of madness. Of course, in Mrs. H's state of grief it did not occur to her that she had called Tom's last name wrong and the ladies had no clue. All the ladies knew was that Tom Selleck had not been to the funeral home while they were present. Remember, Tom Selleck is a movie star. What a hoot! This was a classic case of mistaken identity.

Mrs. P: The Name Tag

Visiting staff at hospice can travel to some remote areas. So it was when visiting with Mrs. P. She lived with her daughter and son-in-law. Mrs. P had very good family support. Well, on one of my visits, Mrs. P's son was visiting from South Carolina. He talked very lovingly about his mother and seemed to be a perfect gentleman. As I was leaving, he walked me to the door and into the yard. When we entered that yard, he seemed to be looking at me strangely. He came closer, and I backed up. Finally, he asked me do you have any vowels in your name. Of course, I stated that I did, because I do. It never occurred to me that he was looking at my name tag.

My name tag read Annie B., LBSW, MSW. He finally asked, "How do you pronounce that… B.LBSW, MSW?" I had to laugh because I really thought the man was looking at my breasts, but he only wanted clarity on what my name was. I explained that the B stood for Brown and the other letters were my professional title, LBSW being Licensed Bachelor Social Worker and MSW being Master Social Worker. I really was on the wrong track that day.

Mrs. C:
The Little White Pill

Laughter is a great spirit lifter. When visiting with Mrs. C, you never knew what you were going to encounter. Mrs. C had a great sense of humor even in the midst of her own diverse struggles. She was unable to walk and she sat in a chair most of the time. Like myself, Mrs. C was overweight and she loved her some angel food cake. The trouble was that she was a diabetic and she did not like following her diet plan, which would have helped her tremendously.

She was also not compliant with her medication most of the time. She actually made a joke of taking her medication when I would ask her was she taking the medication the way she was supposed to. It was on one of these occasions that she told me the most hilarious thing I ever heard about taking medication. This is how the conversation went:

Me: "Have you been taking your medication?"

Mrs. C with a laugh: "You know I have not."

Me: "You know that you need your medication to make you feel better."

Mrs. C: "I do not take that little white pill because since I am so big, the little white pill would get lost because the little white pill would not know where to go."

Never heard anything like that before and have not heard anything like that since. We had these conversations about medication and eating right on most visits as long as Mrs. C was a patient before she made her transition into eternity.

Mr. E:
Television or Reality

When Mr. E came to be a patient of hospice he was an amputee; therefore, it was difficult for him to get around or go outside of the home. Of course,

Mr. E had a wheelchair but he loved to be independent and not use it if he could get away with it. He was a friendly man, but he preferred to stay in his room most of the time when I visited; therefore, most of my time was spent with Mr. E's caregiver.

The times when I visited with Mr. E in his room, he would be smoking and watching television. We all know that watching television can have a positive or negative effect on the mind, especially when that is your past-time. Many times if a person becomes confused near the end of life they relate to things they spent lots of time enjoying. Mr. E was no exception; he became confused near the end. It was during one of my visits near the end of Mr. E's life that he exhibited more confusion than usual. When asking Mr. E had he slept well the night before, he said he had not.

Upon further questioning Mr. E, he stated he did not sleep well because he had visitors the night before. I asked why he did not tell the visitors that he needed his rest and Mr. E replied that he had, but they did not want to go home. I knew that Mr. E was confused, but I asked him anyway who the visitors were. He replied that they were the Robinsons.

Of course I did not know if he actually knew any friends who were Robinsons, but upon returning to the living room, Mr. E's caregiver informed me that no one had visited. I asked her the significance of the name Robinson and the caregiver told me they were the family from "Duck Dynasty," a television show. I had to laugh because I had never heard of the show. After that incident, the same weekend, I found the television show and I watched it and believe me, the show was a hoot. Needless to say Mr. E lost his battle with a terminal illness, but I get to smile when I am in Wal-Mart or any other store and they are advertising products from Duck Dynasty because I remember Mr. E.

Mrs. B:
Beauty Handcrafted

Mrs. B was a remarkable quilt maker. When she came to hospice she had some memory impairments. She, like the lady who used to mimic me, always asked where I had been every time I visited. She would say, "I thought you forgot about me." I would assure her that I could never forget about her. Every time I would visit she would have another pattern for a quilt she was going to make. We had a joke between us that she had homework and that was to finish a quilt before I came back to visit. She never did her homework. She told me stories about when she was rearing her children and how she had to cook so many biscuits and now she does not cook at all. My visits were enjoyable because she had so much beauty to show in her quilts but also beauty in her heart.

Mrs. C:
Have You Ever Heard of Such a Thing?

You have got to love your patients and the things encountered in their homes. Mrs. C was an elderly lady who was bedbound. She was a kind lady with a great sense of humor. She would lie in bed and most times you would think she was sleeping, but she would always answer if you spoke directly to her. I quickly learned she always had her wits about her even though her answers were not always oriented. I had to watch what I said or she would call me on it.

One day, she was not in a talkative mood and I told Mrs. C I guess I would have to go after being there for about 30 minutes and Mrs. C did not say but a couple of words. Well, Mrs. C's daughter and I started another conversation and I made the mistake of saying again that I would be leaving and I said, "Well, I guess I had better go, because Mrs. C is not in a talking mood today." Mrs. C responded with, "Well, you said you were going to go." Mrs. C's daughter and I laughed. That day she was right on it because that is exactly what I said. I learned that even if someone is disoriented on arrival they might just become oriented before I leave.

But the greatest laugh at Mrs. C's home was not even about what Mrs. C might say, but rather about Mrs. C's daughter, who confessed what she observed about her potbelly pig and dog. According to Mrs. C's daughter the pig and the dog had become good friends. On one occasion, Mrs. C's daughter told me that the pig had begun to think that it was a dog and had actually barked. Now you go figure that one out. I cracked up with laughter. I just love my job because I never know what I might hear in a day's time.

Mrs. E:
When a Patient Gets Comfortable

Mrs. E came to us in a pitiful state. She was in lots of pain from her illness, but she also had some bedsores; however, that was not the saddest part of the story. Mrs. E had been in an abusive relationship for many years and she was fearful and did not trust easily. When she seemed to think that someone was going to touch her she would cry out. After weeks of encouraging her and reassuring her she began to get more comfortable with the staff.

What was so beautiful about our relationship with Mrs. E was that she had a birthday during the time she was in hospice. That fearful woman who anticipated pain smiled on her birthday and though she was confused, she had an answer when she was asked how old she was. She said she was fifteen. What was so great about that was that Mrs. E finally was comfortable medically and for the first times in years she was happy.

Hospice care ministers to the total person and in this case to see such a change was wonderful. This is just one example of the rewards of hospice care when physical, emotional, mental, spiritual, and social teamwork makes all the complicated issues worth it to get the victory.

Mr. D:
A Great Imagination

Upon arrival to Mr. D's home, I asked him how was he doing and his reply was, "I am doing without." If I asked Mr. D how he was feeling, he would reply, "With my hands."

So it was with Mr. D. Mr. D was in his nineties and was confused sometimes, but he never seemed to be confused when it came to his imagining he still had it going on sexually at that age.

He had such a sweet wife and she appeared to be embarrassed when I first started coming to visit, because he always tried to tell me that Mrs. D was not treating him right. I would ask him what it was Mrs. D was not doing right and he would reply, "Mrs. D will not put but one foot on the wall." Mrs. D soon got over being embarrassed, because I could always make Mr. D laugh when I would tell him that his and Mrs. D's feet belonged on the floor. Mind you, when he referred to the foot on the wall, Mrs. D would say all he thought about was sex. He had trouble walking and she was so fragile. Nothing like thinking you might have it going on in a sick body that is nearing a hundred. By the way, Mr. D assured me that he was going to live to be a hundred, but he did not make it.

During the course of caring for Mr. D, Mrs. D had a fall that began her downward decline and actually, she never really was the same. She died and Mr. D could not remember most of the time that she was dead, but he still talked about the foot on the wall.

One of the things that I loved about Mr. D was I could also make him laugh. Until the last few weeks of Mr. D's life, he would tell me things that were unbelievable. I asked Mr. D one day what had he been doing and he told me he had been catching frogs. He further said that he was cooking the frogs and they jumped out of the skillet and then out the window. He thought that was so funny because I told him he knew that he had not caught no frogs and tried to cook them. God bless his heart.

Nevertheless, one of the beautiful things he shared with me was that as he was building their home, he allowed Mrs. D to nail one nail in the floor so that she could say that she actually helped to build their home. I hope when he joined Mrs. D that he just gave her a smile and hug and did not want her to put both feet on the wall.

Mr. F:
The Value of Keeping Up with Your Teeth

Mr. F was a fragile little elderly man who was very unhappy with life. My meeting him consisted of him giving me short answers and the attitude of hurry up and go. On one occasion when I arrived, Mr. F was lying on his bed and he was not very talkative that day. I noticed that his dentures were not being worn; one was lying on the bedside table and the other one was on the floor. Well, I mentioned it to him that his dentures were on the floor and I also said the same thing to his grandson. Neither paid me any attention and when one of the dogs in the house came into the room and went over by the bed, I really did not pay the dog any attention.

Well, the grandson came into the room a few minutes later and the dog had gotten Mr. F's teeth. To make a long story short, on another visit I was informed that Mr. F had to have another set of dentures made. After inquiring about what happened, I was told that apparently Mr. F left his teeth lying out and the dog got the teeth again. So I guess the dog thought he might as well try to wear the dentures when he ate. Of course the dentures did not fit, so the dog chewed them up. I thought about my own dentures and what I once heard that your dentures will not fit in anyone else's mouth. But I never would have thought that a dog would try to test out that theory.

Mr. I:
You Don't Have to Have Money to Be Rich

There is a scripture that says that money answers all things. While money is important, there are some things more valuable. So is the story about Mr. I. We admitted Mrs. I to hospice and when I went to conduct my psychosocial, I was greeted by

Mr. I. The first thing that he told me after saying hello was that he wanted to repeat to me what he had told the nurse that came out to admit Mrs. I, and that was he wanted Mrs. I to be taken care of and the rest of the family could take care of themselves.

Well, the house was not very tidy and by the looks of the place, it was obvious that this was a poor family. Even though they may have been poor in earthly resources, Mr. I was rich in love and his pride was intact. He did not believe in handouts. When I visited he made sure that I always had a place to sit that was clean. Mr. I was the kind of person who, if you planned on being a help, then you had to earn his trust and respect. During the time of Mrs. I's stay with us, the family had to move from the house where Mrs. I was admitted. By this time I had learned if I was going to offer to help with any resources, I had to present the resource as "Everyone needs help at some point in their lives," and not as "You do not have anything, so I am going to get you this or the other."

The latter would not have worked with Mr. I; I am sure that he would have asked me to leave and not come back. But treating Mr. I with dignity and respect, I was able to win him over and in the end, I was able to approach him and say, "Mr. I, would you mind if I did such and such for Mrs. I?" and he would agree.

Never was there a time that Mrs. I did not have her bare necessities without my help, but being concerned about the entire family, it was vital to take some of the burden off Mr. I. by assisting him to have what was needed in the home to better make Mrs. I comfortable. The lesson within this lesson was that Mr. I took pride in taking care of his family that he loved and any help granted had to be presented with love and not necessity.

Mr. Z:
Making it to the Finish Line

Talladega County is known all over the country for its contribution to the sport of racing. Racing fans from all across the country come to Lincoln,

Alabama twice a year to be part of the excitement. Personally, I've never been to a race, but I love to see all the beautiful RVs rolling into town. I was close one time to being able to tour the speedway. Mr. Z was supposed to have taken me on a tour, but time did not permit it to be so. Mr. Z had been a racer himself. He loved to talk about his time on the track and it was his desire to visit the track one more time.

So a date was set aside for Mr. Z to introduce me to the world of racing, but as life has it sometimes we can plan but circumstances can unplan. Mr. Z became too ill to make that visit before his death, but he did get to make that last run before being committed into the ground. It was arranged after Mr. Z's funeral that the hearse he was being carried to the cemetery in would make a lap around the track and go through the checkered flag. So it was. What a way to finish a race.

Mrs. P: Getting to a Patient Through Unconventional Means

Mrs. P was a sweet little lady. She did not have any daughters but she had two sons who had taken excellent care of her. In fact she had lived with one of her sons but he died shortly before she became a patient.

Mrs. P had some memory problems. One day when her son went outside, the screen door automatically locked. Mrs. P was sitting in the living room when he left, but when he returned and couldn't get back inside, she did not remember how to unlock the door.

While Mrs. P's son was contemplating how to get the door opened, Mrs. P's nurse came on the scene. And so it was when I arrived a few minutes later, I observed the nurse climbing up and going through the window to unlock the door. We really had the biggest laugh because I said to the nurse can you just imagine a news reporter capturing this story and the headlines reading "Hospice workers will go to any lengths to get to their patients." Mrs.

P's son thought the situation was hilarious also, but the patient never had a clue what was so funny.

Mr. P: New Diagnoses Defined

Sitting at my desk one day, I received a call from a patient who was inquiring about my schedule to visit with him. My plan was to visit the patient the day after he called. During the conversation Mr. P told me that he had two diagnoses. Of course being a social worker, I have some idea of which acronyms are used for diagnoses, but by no means do I know them all. However, the acronyms that this patient was using had never been used in my hearing.

As he talked he first said he had SOS. I was looking at the face sheet for the patient, but what he was saying was not listed, so I asked, "What is SOS?" He laughed and said it was short for "stuck on stupid." Being the professional that I am, I said you are not stupid.

Mr. P really thought that was funny so he said to me, "You really do not know me and I have another diagnosis and have had it since I was born." I was sort of afraid to ask what that diagnosis was, so he went on to tell me he has SKS. After a moment of silence, he said, "Don't you want to know what it is?" By then, I wasn't sure whether I wanted to know or not, so I hesitated but finally said, "What is it?" He informed me that it was a "special kind of stupid." Mr. P seemed to get pleasure from shocking people with his self-made diagnoses. I surely was wordless.

We Honor Veterans

War, like terminal illness, has left many scars of undeniable pain in the lives of people across our great nation. To be able to hear the stories of many of our veterans from various periods of wartime are priceless. The stories depict the reality of what these men and women experienced in a way that a movie will never capture.

I am proud to have had these stories shared with me and have a better understanding of the agony that some of these great military heroes went through for me and to have the liberty as an American to even write about their journey after the wars. Many of these heroes did not return home the way they left and as we know, many did not return at all.

I am so grateful that it is being recognized that not only did some of our military service men/women come home from war to an unappreciative nation, but the psychological damage continues to have lasting effects.

What was once called being shell shocked and battle fatigued is now called Post Traumatic Stress Disorder (PTSD). With any psychological problem there remains a stigma and many military persons will not seek the help that they need.

I have the privilege to be in association with a group of retired military persons who have started a helping ministry for those persons who come home and need help and do not have any idea how to navigate the Veteran system to obtain the medical, as well as monetary, benefits that are due to them. This group is called MAPS which stands for Military Assistance Personal Support.

Since the group started there have been some very positive outcomes for the veterans in St. Clair County where there is now a Veteran Court. What a blessing that veterans are given a chance to go through this court, if they qualify, when their behaviors have gone in the wrong direction with so much pain being a driving force. The use of alcohol and other mind-altering drugs to drown out the pain of their experiences has caused other kinds of issues to arise.

Much time, energy, and monetary sacrifices were made by dedicated men and women who are laboring tirelessly to get help for veterans coming home from Iraq and Afghanistan. Even when fighting their own private battles with emotional/mental scars as well as physical disabilities; these veterans made a vow that our men and women of the military returning home would be provided the resources they so rightly deserve.

Honorable mentions go to Otto Fox and John Carter, who have been instrumental in carrying the vision forward. Physical, mental, emotional, social, and financial issues can be sensitive areas for veterans, but since it has been instrumental in my education about veterans, I thought it was important to share some of what has made my work with veterans effective. Knowledge is power and knowing how to reach a hurting veteran is humbling.

Foremost, when it comes to veterans, a social worker and hospice team need to be sensitive to terminal agitation. Many times as a veteran faces his or her own mortality or imminent death, they also relive the war. Close attention needs to be paid to this, because what appears to be physical, may well be emotional. Not all people who have been in service for our country will exhibit emotional pain at the end of life, but if they do, we need to take time to allow them to work their way through their emotional pain.

If the person does not feel comfortable talking to a social worker or other hospice staff, this is an appropriate time to utilize volunteers who are part of the Vet to Vet program. The Vet to Vet program is a joint effort with hospices and Veterans Affairs to match a patient with a veteran from the same branch of service and time period, if possible, in that patient's journey through terminal illness. The following stories are some of my most precious moments with veterans to date; however, each time a veteran is admitted to hospice, I seek to learn from them.

Mr. X:
Got to Get Closure

Mr. X came to us as a patient from the Veterans Administration Medical Center. He was a nice, happy-go-lucky kind of guy. He had a traumatic event during the time he was serving our country but that event was not as traumatic as some of his life choices. Mr. X went through several high and low periods in his time with hospice. There were several times, due to family dynamics, it was determined that Mr. X should be sent back to the VA Palliative Care Unit. Each time Mr. X went, it was suspected that he would not return home. I went to visit Mr. X on one of the occasions he was at the VA.

What was noted most about Mr. X was that no matter what medications he was given, he seemed to be in terminal agitation. It was finally determined that even though Mr. X was near the end of his life, it was not the disease itself that was causing his symptoms of agitation. Mr. X was experiencing emotional pain from some of his life choices and he needed to find some closure.

On his last return home from the VA, I was able to get Mr. X to open up about some issues that he needed to seek forgiveness for from his spouse. Oh what a joyful day that was when he got his closure and I was able to witness the healing that came to him. Because of that inward healing from seeking forgiveness and reconciliation, Mr. X was able to finally find rest and he died two days later with his family by his side.

Mr. P:
Don't Let it Be Said Too Late

When I wrote in the prior story about terminal agitation concerning one of the veterans that I served, it resulted in a happy ending; however, I remembered another story that involved terminal agitation and the end result was not the same. Mr. P was also a veteran and he experienced terminal agitation, but he was unable to voice what was troubling him because of his diminished mental status. Mr. P would become agitated because he tried so hard to communicate some unresolved issue about his experience in the military.

I mentioned this story because it is my desire for veterans, as well as any other persons, who have issues forgiving or asking for forgiveness to get those issues resolved when you first recognize that there is an issue in your life. Forgiveness has such a healing effect and no one should have to go through emotional pain because of failure to get it resolved.

Forgiveness is a theme/teaching throughout the Holy Scriptures and it is taught in the model prayer that we are to forgive others as God and others have forgiven us. So many times we fail to adhere to the urgency of reconciliation and we ignore the implications of later agony and pain.

So prevalent is this problem that I was inspired to write a book titled, "Christians with Pervasive Issues" a couple of years ago. The book contains some of the issues that people face daily and find themselves pushing the problems into their subconscious to be dealt with at a later time. Regrettably, for many people there is never a good time to address the issues and then it causes undue emotional pain at the end of life. Sometimes the issues go unresolved because people do not know how to get the closure they need. Therefore in "Christians with Pervasive Issues," there is a guide included for victims and perpetrators to find healing from their issues.

Mr. Q:
A True War Hero

Mr. Q sat in a wheelchair; he was paralyzed from his neck downward. He depended on others for transferring from chair to bed and bed to chair. Mr. Q was injured in World War II when he was bombed in a foxhole. Most people would have been bitter and angry, but not Mr. Q; he was a gentle-spirited man with a great sense of humor. He always would playfully tell me that he was not being treated right by his family. And I would reply that I felt so sorry for him. It was just so sad that he received such terrible treatment when he was being loved and adored so much and he would laugh. Laughter was one of the things that made my visits with Mr. Q so enjoyable.

One of my laughing spells that almost had me on the floor came from a joke about the University of Alabama football team. That year, Alabama had a rough year and lost many games and was in the process of looking for another coach. Well, I am not an avid sports fan; therefore, I was not keeping up with what was going on with the search for a coach.

That day when I arrived at Mr. Q's house, he was joking as usual. He asked me had I heard that Alabama had hired a new coach, and of course, I stated that I had not heard. Mr. Q went on to tell me that the University of Alabama had hired either a Chinese or Japanese man. I was buying into it because, as previously stated, I was not up on the news.

Mr. Q finally asked me if I wanted to know what the name of the coach was, and I replied that I did. Mr. Q stated that the new coach's name was "Win-One-Soon." Did you get the joke? He laughed so hard at me because he had pulled one over on me. Of course, there was no such coach. To the credit of the University of Alabama's football team, though, they hired a great coach and went on to win two straight national championships.

Mr. Q did not get to witness the team's winning streak because he became too weak to fight anymore. He died a true hero. In death, he may have surrendered and lost the battle, but he was still a winner when it came to the war.

Mr. K:
Wrong Support Group

Mr. K was a man in his eighties. He had a beautiful home on the lake and seemed to have a comfortable living. Mr. K's wife had died several years before Mr. K became a hospice patient. During discussions with various staff members, it was determined that Mr. K had not allowed himself to grieve the death of his wife.

Mr. K was invited to participate in "grief" support meetings. He inquired about what went on in the meetings and he was educated about the purpose of the meetings. At first, Mr. K declined to come. One day a commotion was heard outside our office and I went to investigate. Mr. K had arrived and the commotion was concerning Mr. K almost running into the building with his van.

At the first meeting, Mr. K was very observant. He barely said anything other than introducing himself. At the next meeting, Mr. K was noticed to be handing out business cards. He had a conversation with one of the women attending the grief support meeting and seemed to be enjoying himself. When I talked to the chaplain, we both thought that coming to the grief meetings was what Mr. K needed.

Mr. K attended another meeting and then he failed to come back again. On one of my visits to Mr. K's home, I asked why Mr. K was not attending the meetings anymore. Mr. K informed me that he did not want to come to the meetings anymore because all the women there wanted to talk about was their deceased husbands.

Well, I stated to Mr. K that at grief support meetings, people talk about their deceased loved ones. Mr. K stated to me that the meetings were not for him, because he had given out his business cards and he had not heard from any of the women. He stated to me plainly that he did not need to talk about his deceased wife and he did not want to hear about the women talking about their deceased husbands. He wanted a girlfriend and he guessed that grief support group was the wrong group to find one at.

Shortly thereafter, Mr. K attended a funeral in his home town and he met up with a lady who was a friend of the deceased family. They talked and do you know what? Mr. K liked this woman and she became his friend. They were able to have lunch a couple of times and talked on the phone. Shortly thereafter, Mr. K died. I guess you don't get too old or sick to need the companionship of the opposite sex. He was a deserving veteran.

Mr. Y:
Small in Stature but Big in Mind

When I think of a man short in stature I often think about the Bible character, Zacchaeus. This man wanted to see Jesus and he could not because he was not tall enough; therefore, he climbed up in a tree to make sure that he could get a glance at Jesus. Zacchaeus was rewarded for his efforts and so it was with Mr. Y. He was short in stature, but he also had a big heart. He lived in a beautiful home with his wife. He was a jolly fellow who always had something funny and nice to say. He loved Jesus and it was evident by his conversations.

Several things come to mind when I think about Mr. Y. I remember so well when I was conducting my psychosocial assessment that I asked Mr. Y if he had served in the armed forces. He replied that he had. Upon further examination, I found out that Mr. Y had served in the Army and was a World War II Veteran. When I asked Mr. Y if he had been in combat, he replied jokingly that he was headed to war, but the Japanese heard that he was coming and they surrendered. It's amazing what a man of such small stature can think of in his mind!!

Another memorable time was when I went to Mr. Y's home and he shared with me some insight he had about the pearly gates that are mentioned in the Bible. After contemplating about the pearly gates, Mr. Y's assessment was that there had to be some very large oysters for them to produce those big pearls to place on the gates in heaven. I never would have thought of such a thing.

Mr. Y was very fortunate to have very good caregivers. Mrs. Y was very serene and as quiet as Mr. Y was noisy. Regrettably, during our time of taking care of Mr. Y, it was found that Mrs. Y had cancer. We took care of them both until their deaths which were several weeks apart. I guess Mr. Y is up in heaven explaining to the other saints about those pearls.

Mr. G:
A Lesson on Returning to Your Youth

Meeting Mr. G came during a difficult time in his life. He was the husband of Mrs. G who had a diagnosis of cancer and dementia and she became one of my patients. She was a very loving lady and she loved her plants and she also had a dog that she loved. Mrs. G fought a good fight, but she lost the battle.

During the time Mrs. G was sick, Mr. G had a severe case of Chronic Obstructive Pulmonary

Disease (COPD) and had difficulty breathing, but he refused to wear oxygen during the day. He continued to drive and he also kept up his yard. Less than a year after Mrs. G's death, Mr. G became a patient. He was just as stubborn as a patient as he was while we were caring for Mrs. G. Mr. G used his age as leverage to dictate what he was going to do or not going to do.

Mr. G was a WWII veteran, and he talked to me about some of his experiences. He told me of a time when there was snow on the ground and the snow was deeper than he was tall. I inquired how he survived the snow and he talked about sleeping down under the snow and eating cold frozen food out of a can. What a sacrifice he made for our country by serving as a solider.

Mr. G loved to garden and I told him that I had decided to plant some seeds to find out if I could grow vegetables. Mr. G was glad to be my teacher, but he refused to not have a garden of his own. He was so determined. Several staff members tried to talk him out of trying to plant a garden, because his medical condition had gotten worse. He did plant some vegetables in pots but he also plowed up a small space to plant. Mr. G's reasoning was that if he had to crawl to plant his garden he was going to do it. He said that he crawled before walking when he came into this world and if he was not able to walk and plant his garden, then he would crawl as he was leaving this world. My lesson was well taken from Mr. G because my vegetables grew and I was able to enjoy some squash and tomatoes, but a greater lesson was that with determination you can do whatever you want, regardless of personal limitations.

Mr. F:
A Pool Shark

I never would have thought that you could find a pool shark at a center for seniors. Mr. F was a patient who had severe problems trying to breathe. He wore his oxygen approximately 23.5 hours daily. Wearing oxygen did not cramp Mr. F's lifestyle, it just gave Mr. F the breath he needed to shoot pool at the senior center and play in the senior's pool tournament.

On the day of the tournament, Mr. F was not feeling his best, but he made the effort to go and play. He did not win, but he was our champion at hospice right on. Mr. F liked to view beautiful websites for special e-mails to send to various individuals but especially to the staff at hospice. On days when I was feeling a little blue I would receive a beautiful e-mail with an attachment from Mr. F. He was a jovial person and seemed to be in a good mood every time I visited.

The doctor did not believe that he would live more than a few months; however, he was a few days short of one year. And just like that person he was, he wanted to celebrate life and a dinner was planned for family and some hospice staff to go to Logan's for his birthday. The dinner did not take place at Logan's, because on the day the dinner was planned, Mr. F's funeral services were held. What a glorious time he must have had dining with Jesus. Glory be to God!

Mr. C:
A Good Neighbor is Always Welcome

Upon admission, it was known that Mr. C did not have a caregiver in the home. Mr. C had a friend who was gracious enough to visit him daily and run errands for him. He had a power of attorney, but the power of attorney was usually not available and lived in another small town. What made Mr. C special was he was a veteran and even though he had a stubborn streak, he was a nice man. Mr. C was proud and was determined to do things on his own and was resistant to having a caregiver in the home. He wanted to stay at home on his own terms.

There came a day when Mr. C was not feeling well at all and the friend who usually cared for him let us know that she would not be able to take on caregiving full time. She continued to make visits and run errands for patient. Mr. C continued to decline and one day it was impossible for him to be left alone.

There were a couple of neighbors who had said they were willing to step in and stay while things were being worked out with a stay at Safe Harbor (Palliative Unit at VA Hospital in Birmingham, Alabama). The neighbor was leaving home, so I flagged him down and asked would he be willing to stay in the home with the patient, and he complied. Don't you just love it when a person says if I can help let me know? That day there was a person who really meant it. As soon as arrangements were made, Mr. C went by ambulance to Safe Harbor and remained there until his death. Thank God that provisions are made for our veterans who served our country and do not always have family to care for them when they are sick.

Mr. T:
Death Comes When Least Expected

Dealing with death and dying is what hospice employees do. However, it is usually expected that the hospice patient will not outlive the caregiver. Not so with Mrs. T. When Mr. T became a patient with hospice, it was expected that Mr. T would not last for a long period of time, but he actually lived months longer. Mr. T was also a veteran who had a wife who took care of him. Mr. T's wife was noted to have some medical issues, but none seemed to be life threatening. Mr. T was almost always in a good mood on visits. He loved to fish.

One day, Mrs. T left home to pick up a relative and she never returned home, because she was killed in a car wreck. Mr. T was devastated at the loss, but he remained stable in his own condition for months. There were several relatives who tried to be Mr. T's caregiver; however, in the end when he did decline, he had to spend his last days at Safe Harbor at the VA hospital in Birmingham, Alabama. Thank God for Safe Harbor and their commitment to taking care of veterans who are terminally ill.

The Young Also Have an Appointed Time with Death

"I am not supposed to bury my child." I have heard this said so many times when a mother or father is facing the death of one of their children. Regrettably, terminal illness does not discriminate when it comes to age. I guess this is one of the areas that cut into my heart the most, because I have children, grandchildren, and now a great-grandchild. It seems so unfair, but when it comes to certain things like dying at an early age, there is no understanding it. It does not seem logical, but it is fair.

I remember reading a book once called "When God Doesn't Make Sense" and it had scenarios where it seemed that some people were in the prime of their lives and that they really had it going on, when suddenly there were a crisis and it totally interrupted what everyone else thought should have been. Some of these individuals were so dedicated and faithful to God, but for some reason, they were not healed in their physical bodies here on earth.

The most valuable lesson I have learned from this is even though the physical body was not healed and it returned to the dust from whence it came, when a person is a Christian they are eternally healed and with our Lord and Savior. There have been times with all the sorrows and pains of life, it makes me a *little* spiritually jealous, because I have to remain here and go through all this craziness we call life and I say God knows best. To be blessed to witness young people go through a terminal illness with grace, humility, and praises to a Mighty God is a treasured gift.

Mr. L:
Oh, How I Love Jesus

Have you ever met a young man who had faith like Job? Well, I was fortunate enough to meet such a young man. This young man was in a battle with cancer and went far and near for treatment. After there was no more treatment available, he became a patient with hospice and I was his social worker. I had heard some interesting stories about this young man's faith before I met him and what I heard did not even prepare me for such a remarkable visit.

Traditionally, social workers are thought to be so professional and stony; however, I do not consider myself to be the norm when it comes to being a social worker. On my first visit, I instantly formed a bond with Mr. L. He was such an anointed young man. Also, he was an avid Alabama football fan. His room was decorated in Alabama colors.

Upon entering the room, I found Mr. L to be very weak in his body, but very strong in his testimony. Actually, he was propped up in bed with pillows. This was another one of those days when professionalism went out the window with me, because Mr. L patted a spot right by him for me to sit. I pulled off my shoes and sat right next to him with my back propped up against the head of the bed.

He started to tell me some of the things that he had gone through during his quest for healing. He had actually gone to a prayer meeting a few nights before and went to the altar, and again asked that God would miraculously heal him. It was what he said to me after he finished that statement that has stayed with me. He said "I am in a win-win situation." He further explained that if God healed his physical body, he could use his testimony to bring others to Christ, but if God did not heal his physical body; then, he would be going home to be with his Lord and Savior.

My heart was so full at the time to hear a twenty-one year old make such a profound statement. He said while he awaited his fate, he wanted to be a living sanctuary for God, because he knew that if God did call him to his heavenly home, to be absent from his physical body was to be present with the Lord.

On the day that Mr. L died, he had been unresponsive and the family was waiting for him to take his last breath. I was blessed to be in the home with our chaplain who was sitting beside Mr. L's hospital bed and the chaplain began to quote, "…to be absent from the body is to be present with the

Lord..." Mr. L squeezed the chaplain's hand and took his journey into eternity. What a departure!

Mr. J:
A Sense of Humor Even in Dying

Mr. J was a nineteen-year-old male who was diagnosed with cancer. He was a special young man who, according to his family, was mischievous most of his life. After various treatments had failed, Mr. J came to hospice as a patient. He had a very loving family and the support of a young lady that showed a strength way beyond her years.

One of the most memorable things I remember about Mr. J was his sense of humor. There was a day when Mr. J was very weak and his parents were anxious about his every movement. Earlier in the day, Mr. J's parents had eaten something with garlic in it. They were hovering over Mr. J and Mr. J's speech was barely audible; therefore, his parents had to get real close to hear what he had to say. It was apparent that Mr. J was in some discomfort and his parents wanted to know what they could do for him. Mr. J's reply was "Let me breathe." Evidently the smell of the garlic was taking his breath. According to Mr. J's family he had been a rebellious teenager; however, Mr. J received Christ in his life and he had a glorious departure from this world on Easter.

Memorable Conversions

One area of hospice that many people find rewarding is the spiritual aspect of being part of the process of one being lead to God at the end of life. As hospice workers who believe in eternal life, it is important to us that a person comes to know the risen Savior before taking that last breath. We have to lay aside our own theology and embrace who a person is or what they believe on admission.

First and foremost, we pray that there will be time to earn the trust and respect of the patient/family to lead them to Jesus, if they do not already know Him. In hospice people come from all walks of life; therefore, they have all kinds of belief systems. We are not in the home to get the patient to believe all we believe as a Christian, but we do want them to have the fundamental concepts of believing that Christ was born, died and He rose on the third day, and that if you believe that Jesus is Lord you can be saved according to the Scriptures.

Two of my most memorable conversions were men. The first was a very likeable man who professed to be of Jewish background and he was married to a lady who professed to be a Jehovah's Witness. One day while I was in the home, it was brought to my attention that there were some concerns about if the patient died would he be with Jesus. I understand that only God knows a person's heart; however, every person knows if they have truly given their heart to God.

This man I will call Mr. N. Mr. N had a great decline and I was visiting with him. He seemed to be distant on this visit and I asked him if he had some concerns. Since his prognosis was poorer than when we first met, I knew that it was important; if he had not accepted Christ, I needed to try to reach him.

There was no time to beat around the bush, so I asked Mr. N. if he had any pain and he patted his chest. To clarify if it was physical, I asked, "Is your heart hurting?" He indicated his heart was hurting but not from physical illness; however, there was a deep pain. So then I asked, "Do you have some issues that you need to clear up in your heart?" and he looked up at me and spoke the word "angel." I asked if he needed to talk to a rabbi and he shook his head, "No." I also asked, "Do you want me to lead you to the Lord?" He hesitated.

Now even in his critical state he was not ready to accept being led to the Lord by a woman; therefore, I asked him if he wanted the chaplain to come and Mr. N did. The rest is history, because the chaplain came and he led Mr. N to Christ and he died shortly thereafter.

The other story is about a man who considered himself a Buddhist. When I met Mr. I he was kind, but he was difficult to care for because of his belief system. He had all these plans to take care of end of life issues, but time did not seem to want to cooperate with his timetable. Mr. I was suspected to have metastatic cancer to the brain. He shared many things about his life; however, almost everything he told me was opposite of what was true. He said he had two sons and actually, he had two daughters. He denied having any other family, but in the end it turned out that he had siblings and his mother was living, also.

The most amazing thing was that Mr. I would not take his medication, because he said that even though he was not a practicing Buddhist, he could not put all those chemicals in his body for pain. His rationale was that he was in pain because of some choices he had made at various stages in his life and that the pain was his punishment. Mr. I did not have a caregiver in his home, so he wound up having to be placed in an assisted living home. It was during this time that some monks visited with Mr. I and according to those who were present, he gave his life to Christ.

The moral of these two stories is that no matter whom people say they serve as a god, it is important that they get introduced to the Lord Jesus Christ. We never know who will be present when the person accepts the invitation to give their life to Christ, but we have to make every effort to present the Gospel to them.

Part III

- ✓ Annie's Personal Rewards for Serving
- ✓ A Prayer I Will Not Soon Forget
- ✓ My Heart's Desire

Annie's Personal Rewards for Serving

The rewards of ministering to end of life patients are endless. The lessons learned are valuable and has made me a more productive person in society. I have found that some of the greatest teachers in and of life are not in the classroom but are in their homes either in a wheelchair or bedbound. I would like to share three important lessons.

LESSON ONE: I gave my time but they gave me a testimony. Seeing a person go through suffering and many telling me I know I am dying has made me more appreciative of whatever state I am in at this stage in my journey called life. Even though, I have faced many trials/tests and have been an overcomer, my life lesson teachers (my little people) have shown me through their bravery and their vulnerabilities that to be strong does not mean you do not allow your emotions to show. So many times in the past, I have suppressed my emotions when I should have allowed myself to feel whatever it was that I was feeling without condemnation. In the words of Kirk Franklin, "we all hurt and we all feel pain" and we should be allowed to share the bad as well as the good things we experience in life.

LESSON TWO: I provided emotional support; however, they had already been supporters; therefore, they had solid foundations and helped me to build thereon. I take from this walk with my little people the value in having a viable support system in every aspect of life. Sometimes just knowing that we need others is a big step in healing. A slogan from the military is "It takes courage to ask for help." So many people suffer alone because they feel that no one understands what they are going through. Believe me I have been there. Sometimes just saying I don't always have it together to another person in the same situation helps bring another perspective to light as we are able to share that we understand. I remember someone telling me once to always allow another person to tell their story because no matter how small the contribution, everyone has something to bring to the table. Knowing this helps me to develop a personalized care plan for each patient, because there is no set formula.

I guess the most profound of the lessons has been...

LESSON THREE: which is, as they faced death, I learned to live. Being thankful for the things that I so often took for granted have become so important. Making certain I tell my loved ones I love and appreciate them is so vital when we see each other or talk to each other on the phone.

Most of all, I do self-examinations to make sure that I am walking with Jesus daily and giving

Him the glory and praise. This is my number one priority because hearing the stories of my patients made me realize that there is no magic formula to predict when a devastating diagnosis will be given to me or anyone else. With that diagnosis, unless a mighty miracle from God does takes place, the prognosis will be death.

We never know when we might become the one who will need the services that I now provide. It is an honor to be used by God to provide a bright spot in patients' and their families' lives when they are the most vulnerable and need encouragement just to make it through the next few hours because sometimes that is all the time they have left. So I give praise to God for allowing me to experience the losses (death of loved ones) that I used to be so bitter about because when I put aside my notes or my role as a social worker and say I have been a caregiver or I have walked in similar shoes, then I am recognized as someone who can show compassion for the situation instead of someone who is visiting because I am part of a care team.

Not that I understand what another person is going through, because each person's family/friend dynamics are different, but the person who is suffering is more comfortable with sharing because, as someone may say, "Been there and done that." Experience goes a long way in dealing with death and dying, but the most valuable of gifts is having an intimate relationship with God and being sensitive to God's leading as you and I minister/serve those in need of hospice care. Let us not ever take for grant good health.

A Prayer I Will Not Soon Forget

Upon arriving at Mr. X's home, I never would have thought I would leave a different way from how I came. Mr. X was a thin man and appeared to be unkempt. It was my first time meeting him, so I definitely did not know what to expect. He seemed to have his guard up as he talked about how people claim they want to care for you, but they really don't.

Mr. X shared that he had a good work life but he had come off his job for retirement at age sixty-two. He was very candid about making mistakes and regretting some of his choices. There were period of time when Mr. X was forgetful or appeared confused. He said he was not eating because food made him sick. He was living in a little RV camper and there was not much moving room.

When Mr. X sat down he told a story about fishing in heaven. He said he would love fishing to catch some Rainbow Fish, but he said they are so beautiful that he would not be able to stand it if he had to kill them for food. We laughed as my visit was coming to a close. When I stood up, Mr. X requested me to sit back down for a minute. I thought he had something to show me, but what he actually did took me by surprise. He turned and kneeled down on his knees and said the most unselfish, endearing prayer that I have ever heard anyone pray for me.

My heart was so overwhelmed with the earnest petition for my protection, my home, traveling mercies, provisions for any needs for me, my family, and the patients I visit. I left there feeling so blessed and with a new determination to be the best social worker that I can be because Mr. X said he could see the sincerity in me, wanting the best for my patients.

My Heart's Desire

Wanting the best for those who are sick, especially those who have been put in my path, is a daily challenge that I would be able to be of comfort and support to them. It takes denying yourself to get the right answer to the questions: "What can I do today to make someone's life better?"

I must stay prayerful and seek the wisdom that comes from God as I use the skills and resources available. I must continue to avail myself to education. I have been successful in winning most battles, but the war is not over. As long as there is life as we know it, there will be death also. So my journey continues and I look forward to sharing with the world the experiences that are still before me. Until the second part of this project is written my prayer is:

Gracious Father,

I look to you for guidance in my everyday endeavors.

Teach me, Lord, how to go in and out among all kinds of people and teach me how to judge between right and wrong. Help me make the wisest decisions that apply to each patient and their unique situations. I praise you for these past ten years in the vineyard of hospice and I pray that you would keep hospice agencies and all its affiliates safe and secure in your love and provisions.

In Jesus' name, Amen.

About The Author

Annie Clara Brown is a licensed social worker who holds a Baccelerate of Social Work (BSW) from the University of Montevallo and a Master of Social Work (MSW) from the University of Alabama.

Her concentration in graduate school was children, adolescences, and families. Prior experience in the social work field includes: internships at Talladega County Department of Human Resources in Adult Protective Services, and the Cheaha Mental Health Center.

Ms. Brown acquired training through the Alabama Department of Human Resources as a Family Preparation Specialist and training through the Alabama Department of Public Health as Case Manager for Diabetics and Asthmatic persons. She currently works as a hospice social worker with

Lakeside Hospice in Pell City, Alabama. Ms. Brown is responsible for conducting psychosocial assessments, counseling patients and their families about end of life issues, helping patients and their families to access community resources, and conducting grief support groups as needed.

Ms. Brown also works in collaboration with the Department of Veteran Affairs educating staff, community, and other veterans about the Vet to Vet Program. Other interests include working with veterans who suffer from Post-Traumatic Stress Disorders (PTSD) and Traumatic Brain Injuries (TBI).

Ms. Brown is a mother, grandmother, and a great-grandmother. She is also a licensed minister in the AOH Church of God, Inc. She serves as secretary in her local church and is a District Sunday School Superintendent. Ms. Brown is an avid reader. She is a published author of two other books, *Christians with Pervasive Issues* and *Who I Be*.

www.ingramcontent.com/pod-product-compliance
Lightning Source LLC
Chambersburg PA
CBHW071416210526
45465CB00001B/412